Healthy Children
Healthy Lives

How to Raise Kids with Healthy Habits

Sherrie Le Masurier

Healthy Living Tips for Kids (and Parents)

A 'Raising Healthy Kids' Book

ISBN-13:
978-1482345667

ISBN-10:
1482345668

Table of Contents

Introduction

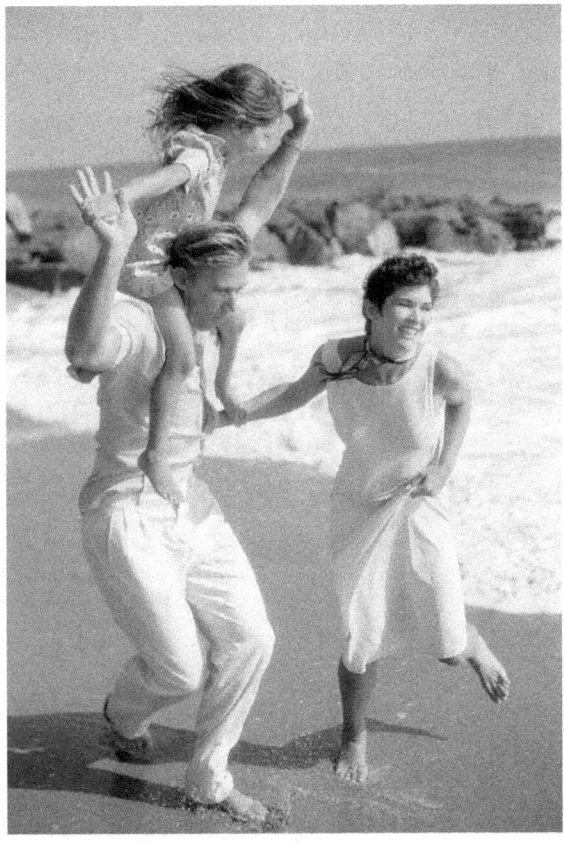

Welcome to **Healthy Children Healthy Lives: How to Raise Kids with Healthy Habits**, a quick-to-digest guide of healthy living tips for kids *(and parents)*.

This healthy habits book is an overview of the types of daily habits that are important to encourage at a young age.

You'll learn tips for maintaining a healthy fitness level, getting adequate sleep and ways to improve your child's eating habits.

In addition to discovering good healthy living tips, you'll find ideas for making lifestyle changes as a family.

One of the best ways to encourage healthy habits is to model them yourself; and the simple and straightforward ideas in this book will help you do just that.

Please note: subsequent books in this 'Raising Healthy Kids' series will explore physical fitness, sleep and nutrition in greater depth.

Sherrie

Making 'Healthy' a Daily Habit

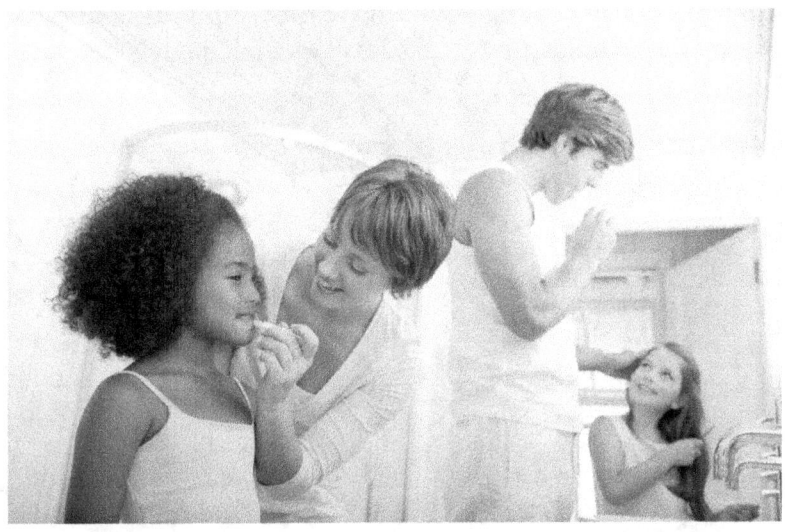

Raising healthy kids is simple right? We provide our kids with nutritious foods encourage physical activity and enforce a regular bedtime and all should be good. The reality is it's easier said than done.

No matter how health-conscious we are as parents, our children have to compete against a number of unhealthy temptations. The fast paced society in which we live also plays a significant role in supporting unhealthy habits in addition to healthy ones.

One unhealthy reality is the ease and availability of fast food whether it's from a drive thru or a box of processed food you pull out of your freezer. Both do little more than lay the groundwork for a lifetime of serious health problems.

Not to mention, contributing to the high percentage of childhood obesity.

With life as busy as it is, how can we raise our kids not only eat right, maintain a healthy fitness level, get adequate sleep but also be healthy and happy?

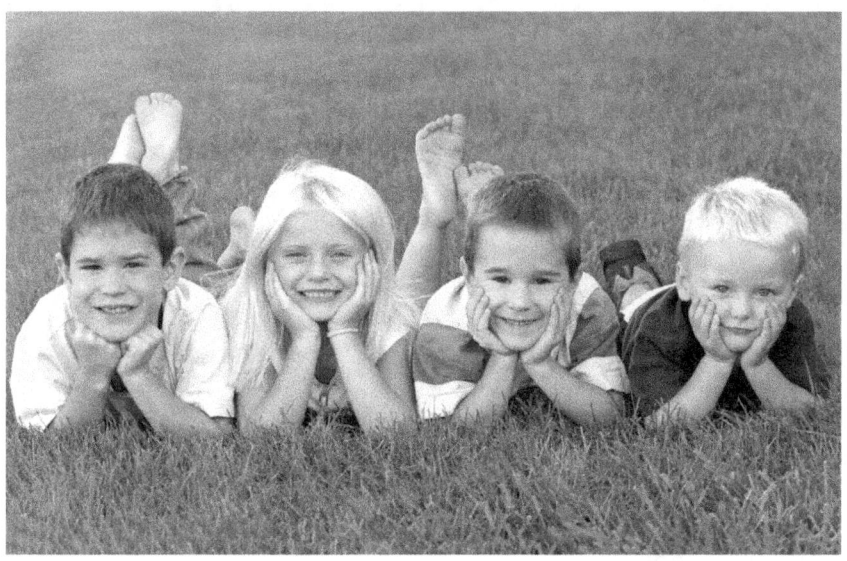

Following are tips to help busy families make healthy habits a part of everyday life.

Keep your kids active

Kids and teens should be active for at least one hour each day. Ideally part of this time is spent outdoors. Encourage activities that raise breathing and heart rates and those that strengthen muscles and bones.

You can easily inject more physical activity into your daily life simply altering the way you do things; like when going for a walk, take your toddler out of his stroller more often. Other ideas include playing hopscotch while waiting for the bus or racing to the end of the road/driveway to pick up the mail.

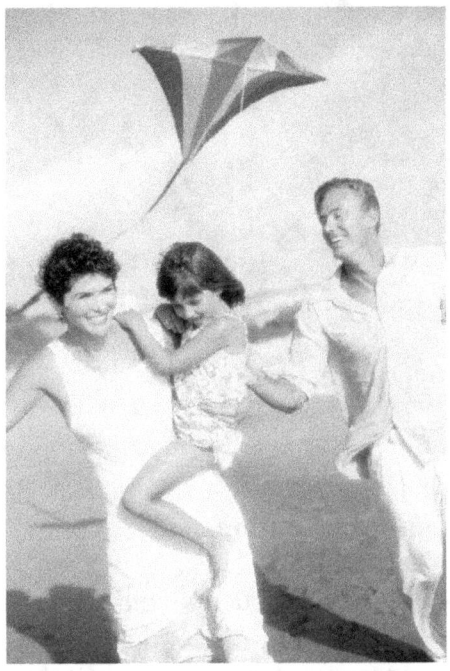

Make lifestyle changes as a family

One of the best ways to improve your kids' habits is to make lifestyle changes as a family with an emphasis on wellness over weight. While weight can be a huge factor, implementing a healthy lifestyle is by far more important, at least initially.

Living healthy as a family is a group effort and doesn't single out any one family member. If we aren't willing to make an overall change to our lifestyle how can we expect our kids to?

Talk about the lifestyle changes you want to make as a family and then implement a few new things each week.

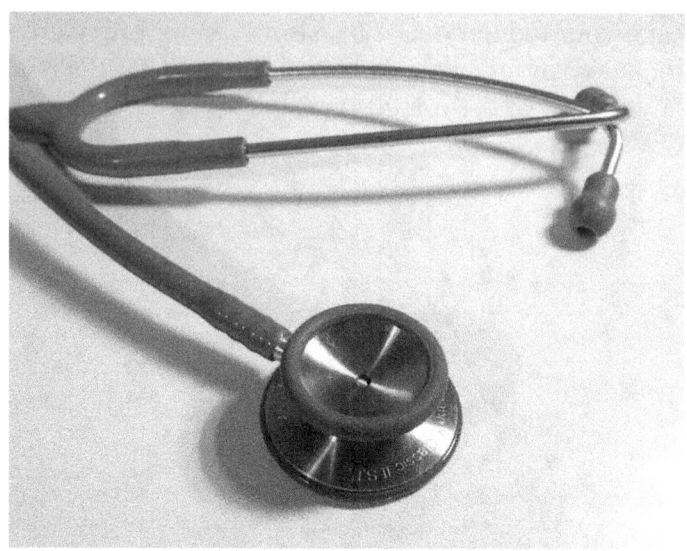

Get check-ups and vaccinations

Routine check-ups, including dental and eye exams, are among the best ways to be proactive and to identify any health issues early on when chances for treatment are better.

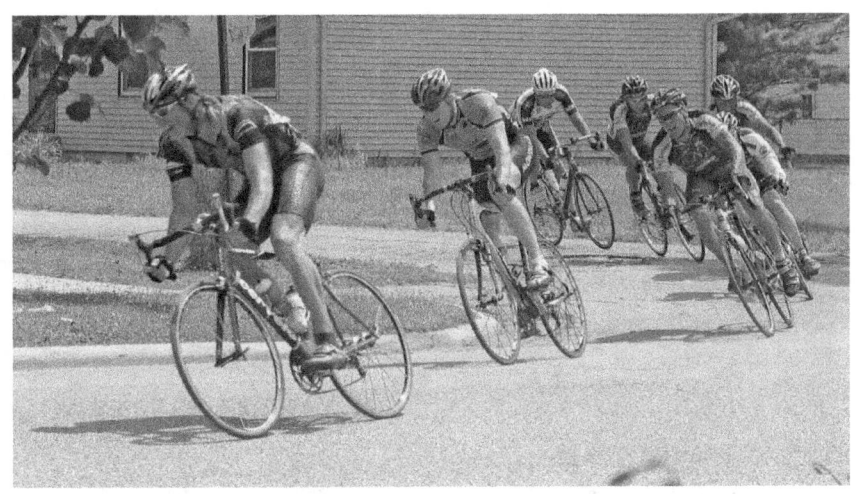

Encourage healthy habits

Help your make safe and healthy choices everyday by setting
positive examples. By modelling healthy habits we show our
children that actions like fastening their seat belts, wearing
helmets, applying sunscreen, brushing teeth, and frequent hand
washing are healthy habits.

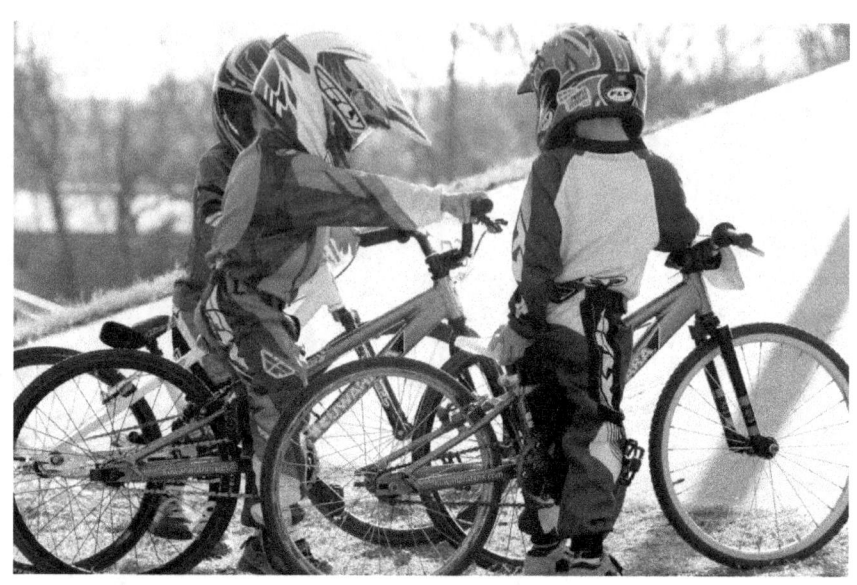

Provide love, support and guidance

Ultimately kids need love, support and guidance. Raising healthy kids takes patience, understanding and know-how. Having an open dialogue about healthy habits and how to make wise choices helps us raise our kids in a safe, loving, and secure environment.

Keeping Your Kids Active

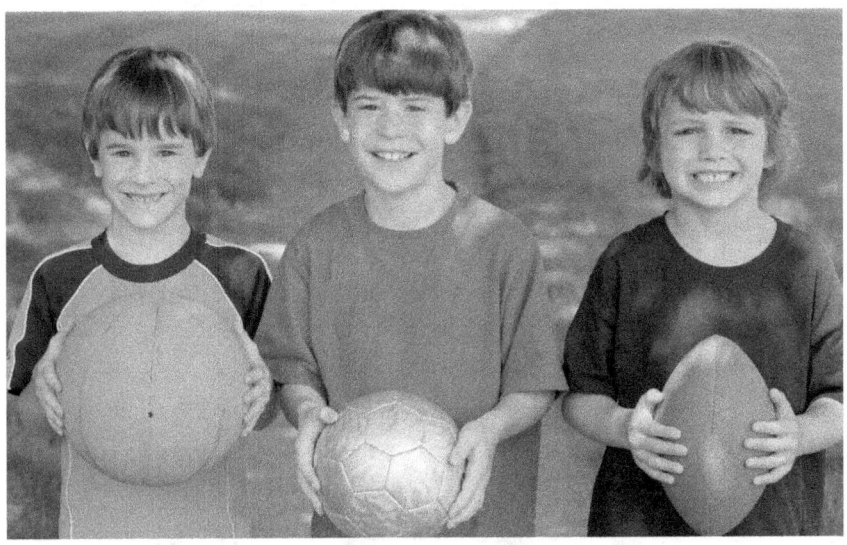

Kids are more likely to succeed if they're healthy and active. As parents we can play a big role in shaping our children's attitudes towards physical activities. While the ultimate goal is to have our kids physically active for at least an hour a day, you may be surprised just how easy it is for your child to stay fit when he finds an activity he enjoys.

Fortunately, many physical activities fall under more than one type of activity, making it possible for kids to participate in many different types of physical activity in a single day. For example, if your son is on a basketball team and practices with his teammates regularly, he's doing both a vigorous-intensity aerobic activity as well as an activity that strengthens his bones. Likewise, a daughter who takes gymnastics lessons is combining muscle and bone strengthening with a moderate-intensity aerobic activity.

The key to raising fit and active kids is to encourage them to participate in activities that are age-appropriate, enjoyable and offer variety.

In addition to aerobic activity, you want to encourage regular activities that strengthen your child's muscles and bones at least three days a week.

Following are some good ways to encourage your kids to participate in informal active play and to get them involved in organized sports activities.

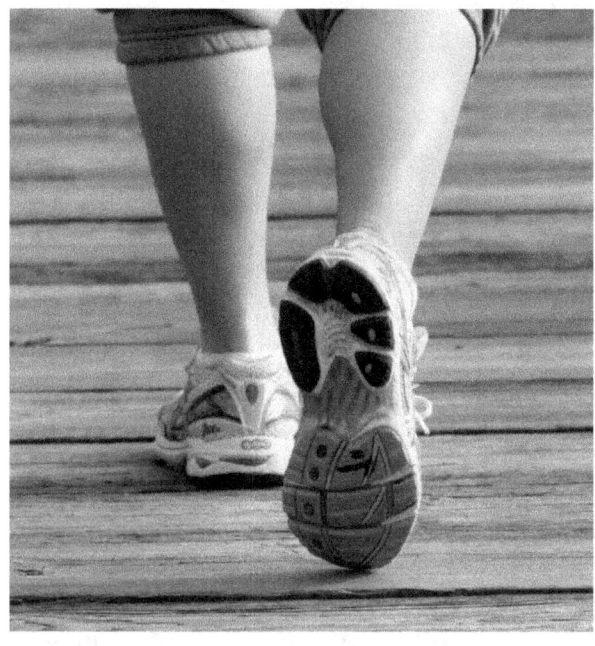

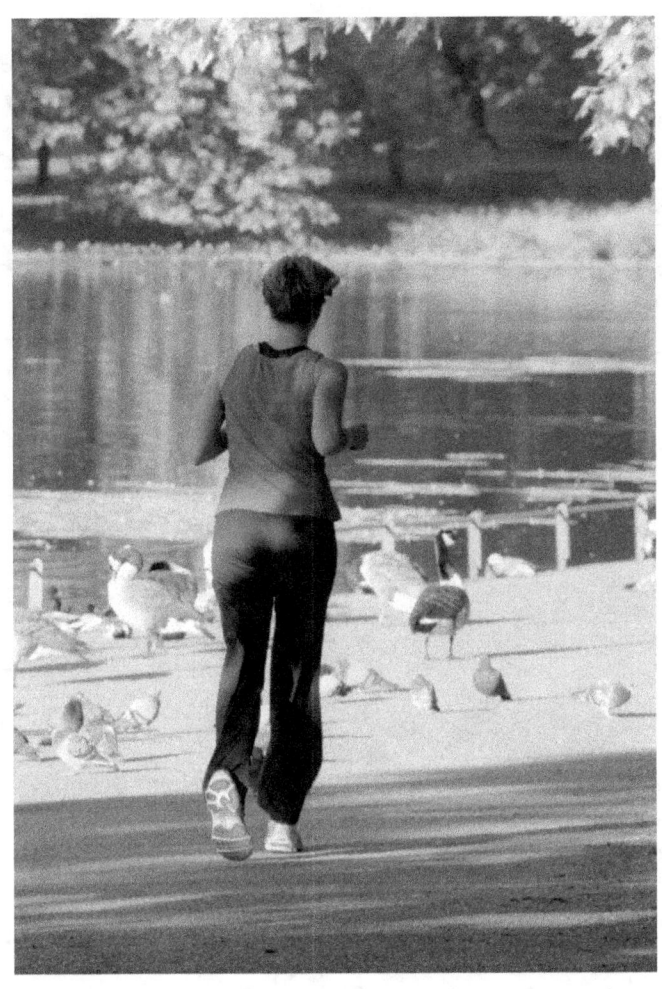

Lead by example

Set a positive example by leading an active lifestyle yourself. Play sports and/or demonstrate a commit to a fitness activity like running or working out at a gym on a regular basis.

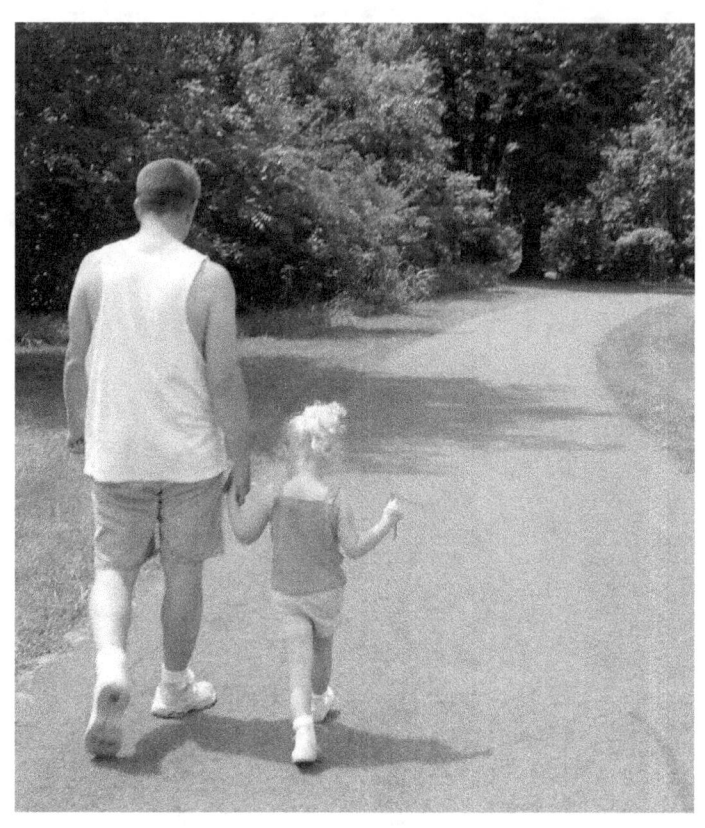

Make physical activity part of your family's daily routine

Take family walks or play active games together.

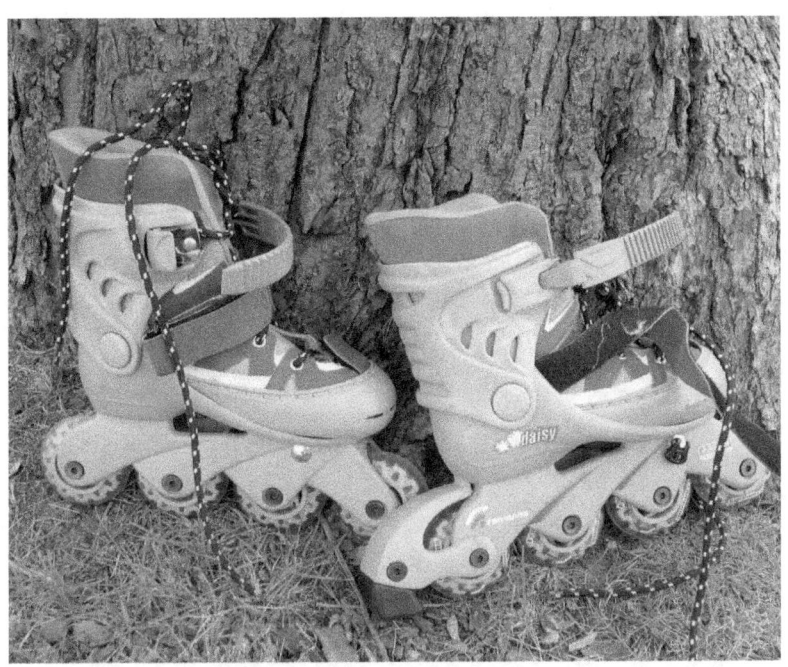

Supply your kids with the right equipment

Encourage physical activity by giving sports related equipment like balls, Frisbees, inline skates etc. as holiday and birthday gifts.

Offer up the right setting

Set the stage for activity by taking your kids to local parks and community fields, and courts for baseball, basketball, and tennis. Testing out new sports and activities as a family is a great way to spark your child's interest.

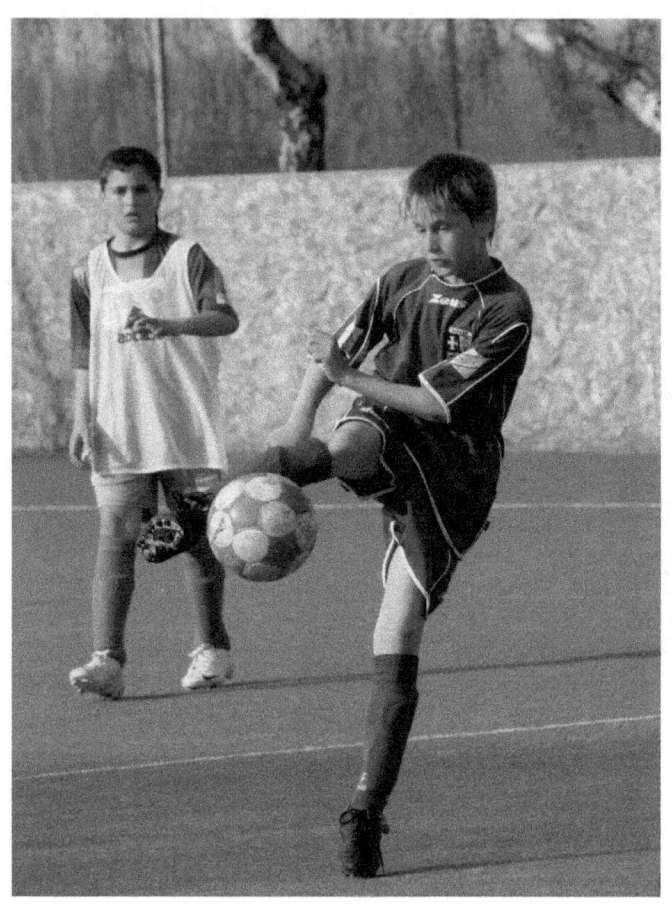

Suggest new activities and offer up encouragement

Encourage your child to try new activities by being positive and supportive of the activities he is good at.

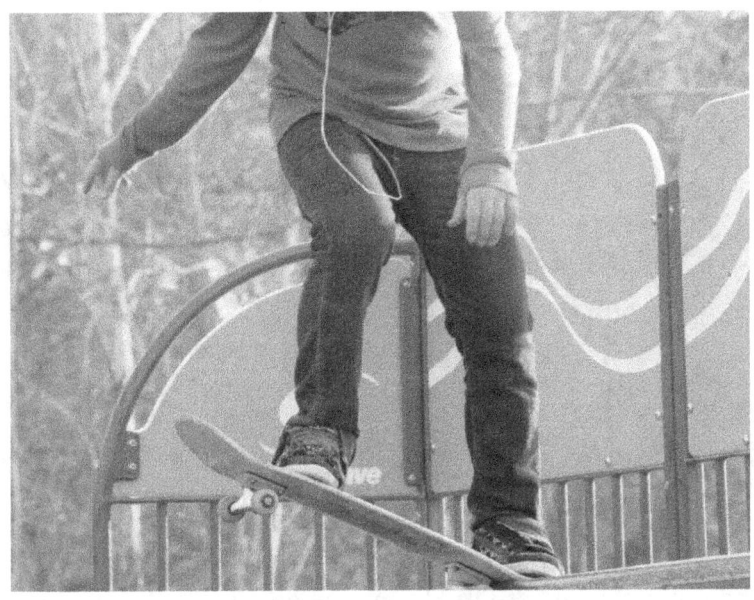

Make physical activity fun

The activities your children participate in can be anything they enjoy. Activities don't have to be structured. Kids can benefit greatly from down time activities that involve a combination of aerobic activity and body strengthening. Encourage activities your kids can do on their own or with friends and family like rollerblading, jogging, or cycling.

A final factor to consider when encouraging kids to get active is whether or not a particular activity will stimulate your children, making it an unwise activity to be done later in the evening.

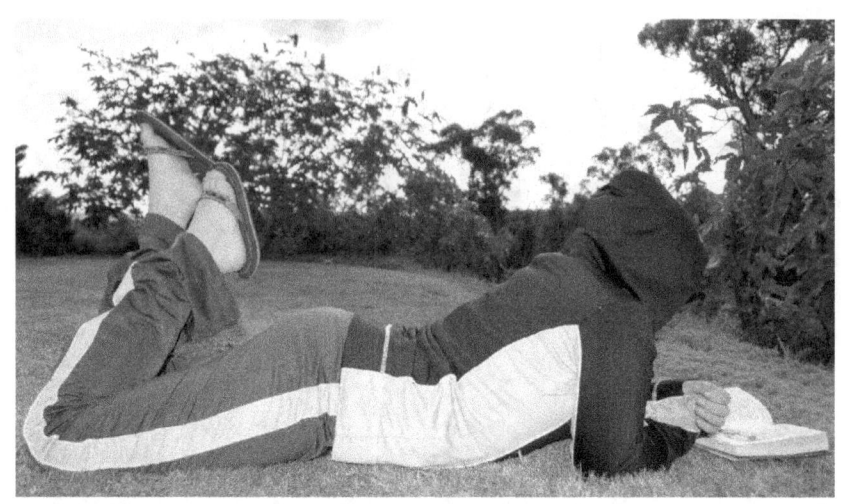

Although physical activity during the day is healthy for sleep, our children's bodies need time to cool down after exercise. Similarly, their minds need time to settle down after activities that require deep concentration. In addition, the stress of performing well may keep our kids from falling asleep easily, when they play sports too close to bedtime.

Getting Enough Sleep

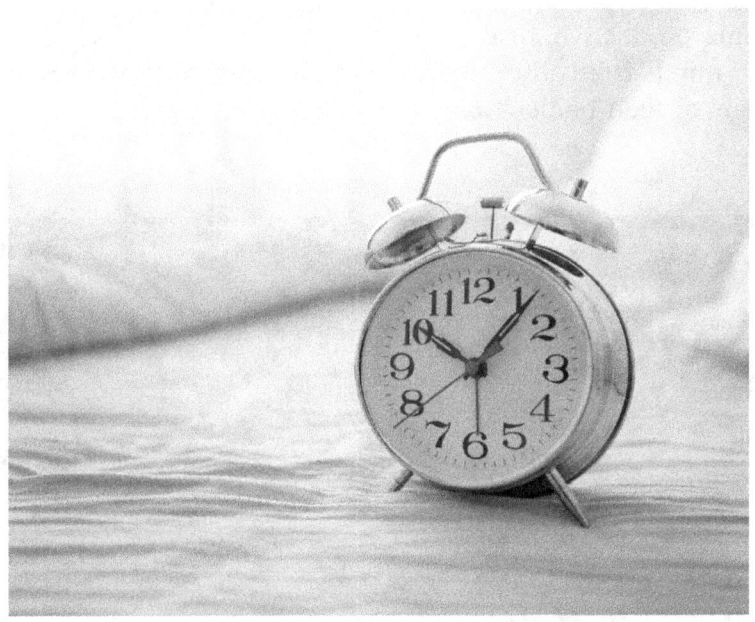

If your kids are yawning and drowsy throughout the day, it's not surprising. An estimated 60 to 70% of students are sleep deprived.

There are no two ways around it - kids need sleep and plenty of it. Our kids' health, emotions, memory, and academic potential depend on it. Unfortunately sleep insufficiency in youth is on the increase, affecting cognitive ability, and your child's emotional and physical well-being.

Just as nutrition and exercise are important factors in raising healthy kids, so are positive sleep habits.

A healthy child is one who can perform his best physically, mentally and emotionally. As parents, we need to prioritize the sleep requirements of our children. We also need to recognize that allowing our kids to put off sleep to study, practice a skill, or hang out with their friends via social media is counterproductive. Insufficient sleep may in fact be preventing their minds from absorbing the information we want them to retain, or their bodies from developing as they should.

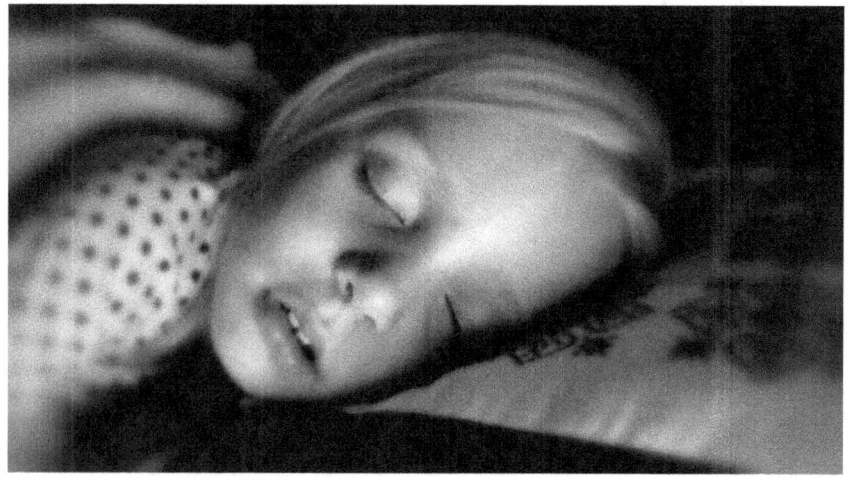

So how do busy families best address this growing problem? Most sleep experts say it starts with consistent bedtime rituals.

While your child's individual needs may vary, the National Sleep Foundation recommends kids get the following hours of sleep: toddlers, 12 to 14 hours; preschoolers, 11 to 13 hours; school-age children, 10 to 11 hours; and adolescents, nine to 10 hours.

Ideally, good sleep 'hygiene' begins when your child is an infant. That said it's never too late to get your child's nocturnal patterns back on track.

Develop a pre-sleep routine

Young children may benefit from routines that include a light snack, a bath and reading before bed. As your children grow, they will associate these positive behaviours with sleep.

Be firm with bedtimes

Kids will try just about anything from starting a battle with a sibling, requesting a glass of water, to having you check their closets or under their bed for monsters, in order to stay up longer.

Defuse the battle, get your child a glass of water, and ward against monsters with a mist. *(Fill a spray bottle with water and add a 'Monster Be Gone' label.)* We may not be able to eliminate our children's resistance to sleep but we can be firm and keep bedtime routines as consistent as possible.

Never use later bedtimes as a reward

Rewarding good behaviour with a later bedtime isn't a good idea. Instead of allowing your child to stay up for 'one more show', record the program for him to enjoy the next day.

Move bedtime backwards

An overtired child will benefit from having his bedroom time moved back 15 minutes every other night until he starts to wake up feeling refreshed.

Get technology out of the bedroom

At night make your child's bedroom a tech free zone – no TV, cell, or computer. Create a buffer by making it a rule that all technology-driven devices are shut off an hour before bedtime.

Keep bedtime snacks light

While sending your child to bed on an empty stomach isn't good, neither is loading them up with a heavy meal. Aim for a balance. Likewise, avoid foods and beverages that act as stimulants e.g. ice cream or chocolate milk.

Nutrition and Healthy Eating

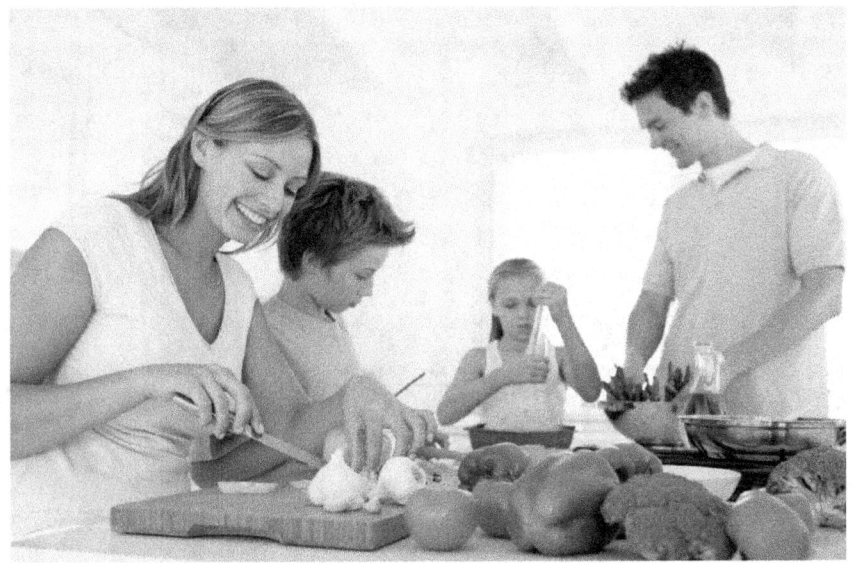

As children grow their nutritional needs change. While we want to encourage proper nutrition, getting our kids to eat the right foods can be a challenge.

In addition to promoting healthy eating habits, the foods we serve our kids will help them maintain a healthy weight and reduce the risk of chronic diseases later in life.

When kids understand why certain foods are healthy and have parents who take the time to teach them how to make healthier food choices and how to cook, they are more likely to make proper nutrition a priority.

Encourage healthy eating and proper nutrition with the following.

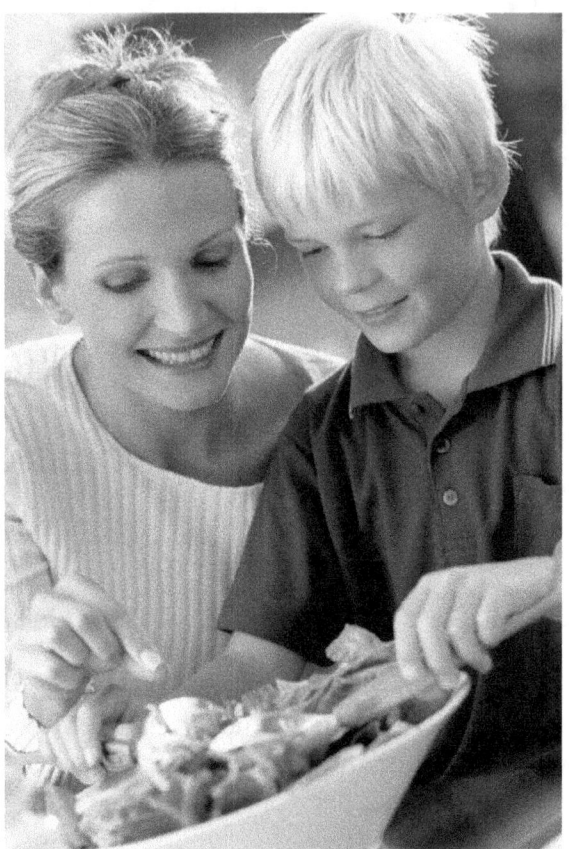

Teach your children how to make wise food choices

Show them how to limit foods high in sugar, fat and sodium by comparison shopping for more nutritional options. Guide your children through the process of buying, preparing and enjoying healthy foods by taking them grocery shopping and seeking their help in the kitchen.

Don't cater to your picky eater

Selective eating and weight problems often go hand in hand.
Don't fall into the trap of buying unhealthy foods just because
it's all your child will eat and whatever you do, don't give up
on introducing new foods. Studies have shown that some
children will eat a new food only after tasting it five or more
times.

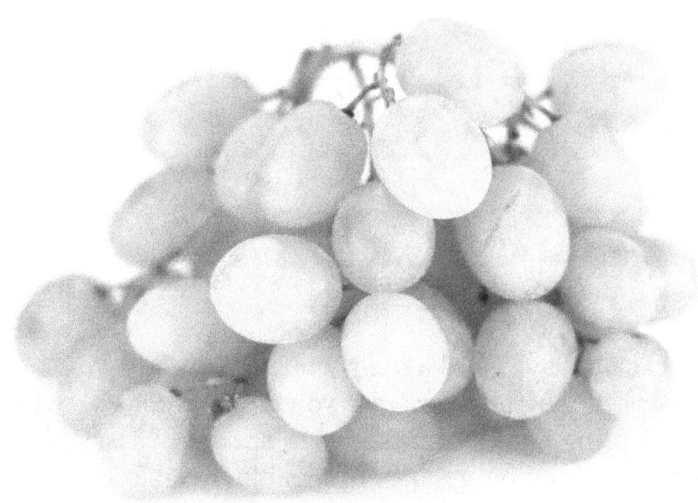

Keep a healthy supply of snacks on hand

The more you serve up fruits and veggies *(and eat them
yourself)*, the greater the chance your kids will too. While it
takes a little extra effort, keeping containers of cut-up fruit and
veggies front and centre in your fridge can really pay off.
Likewise, keep cheese sticks, yogurt, nuts and popcorn *(hot air
popped)* on hand for quick and easy snacking.

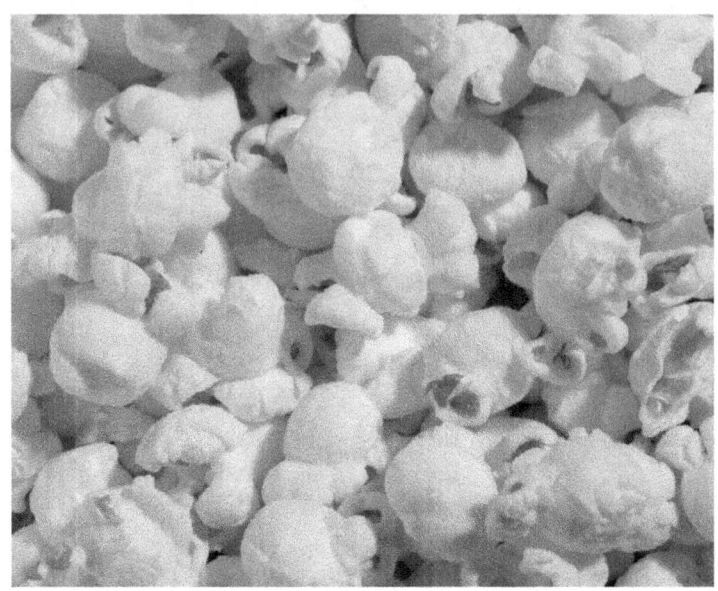

Don't stock unhealthy foods

While you can't always ward against unhealthy foods your child may seek in the outside world, you do have control over the foods you bring home. Limit treats to special occasions and be creative by seeking out recipes for healthier versions of favorite foods.

Serve fluids that fuel

Fluid intake is important, not only the amount we drink but also the quality. You can't underestimate the benefits of keeping your kids hydrated as well as avoiding sugar and caffeine laden beverages.

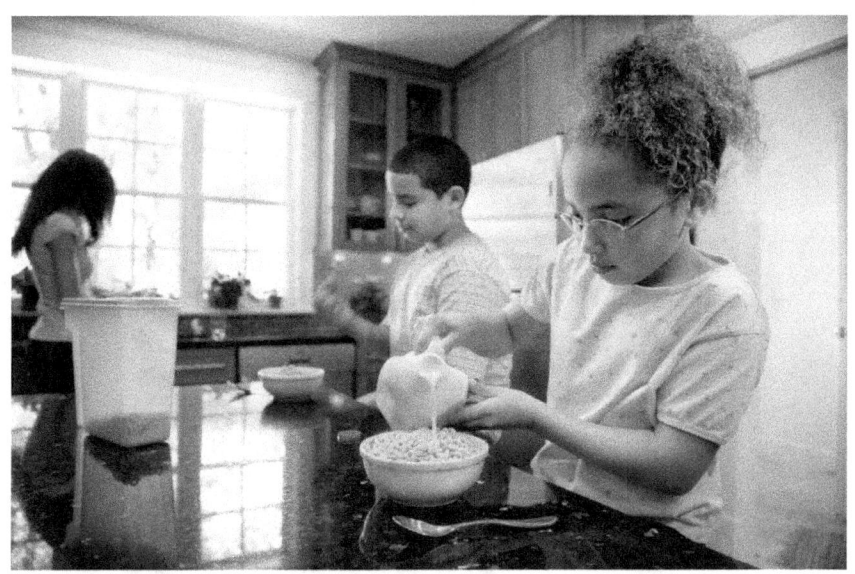

Encourage a healthy breakfast

For kids, breakfast really is the most important meal of the day. In addition to providing fuel for their brain to learn, breakfast will help them maintain a healthy weight. Kids who skip breakfast are also more likely to eat larger, less healthy meals later in the day.

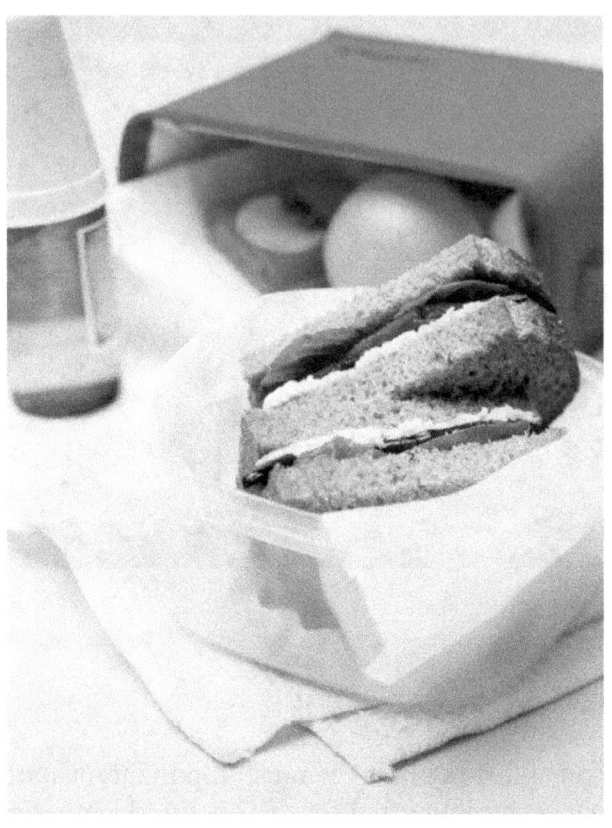

Give your kid's lunchbox a makeover with healthy substitutions

Add variety and more nutrition to school lunches with creative substitutions like using avocado *(add a little lemon or lime juice to prevent discoloration)* or yogurt as a spread instead of butter or mayonnaise.

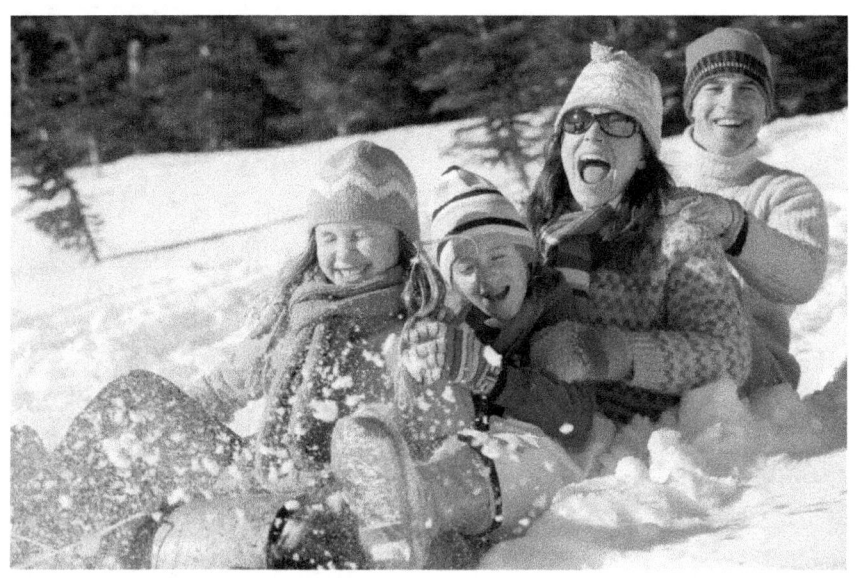

Don't offer up food as a reward

While it's nice to enjoy a treat from time to time, rewarding your children with unhealthy foods on a regular basis can be counterproductive and could lead to nutrient deficiencies, dental issues, obesity etc. Alternatively, sit down with your kids and come up with a list of fun 'activity' ideas for rewards e.g. tobogganing.

About the Author

Sherrie Le Masurier is a professional organizer, decorating consultant, and lifestyle writer who helps parents better organize their home and family life.

To learn more about Sherrie and how she can help you better organize your home and family life, visit www.sherrielemasurier.com where she offers up smart solutions for busy families.

For a complete list of books by Sherrie Le Masurier visit Sherrie's Author page on Amazon.

www.ingramcontent.com/pod-product-compliance
Lightning Source LLC
Chambersburg PA
CBHW070406290526
45790CB00004B/1648